A.C. WELLNEY

FITNESS FOR Streamers Sitters and Gamers

Building Fitness Into Your Daily Patterns

This book was professionally typeset on Reedsy.
Find out more at reedsy.com

Contents

Introduction

Who is this for?

People who stream, sit (working), and game for longer periods of time

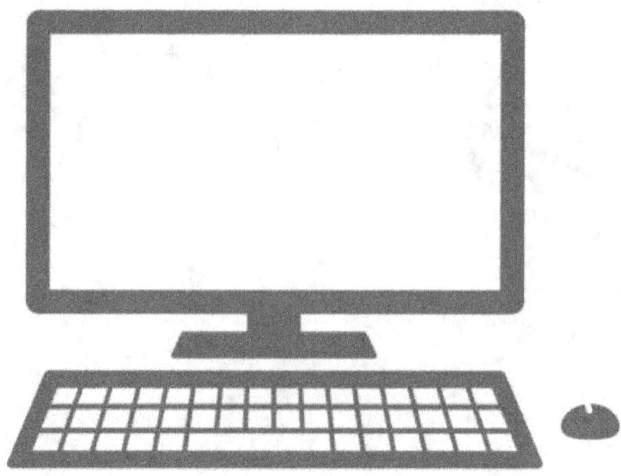

People who are fine with how their body looks and aren't looking to bulk or build muscle

People who don't know how to "hop into a routine" or "fitness" program, but would some day like to get there… or not.

People who would consider themselves lazy or potentially unable to commit to something fully.

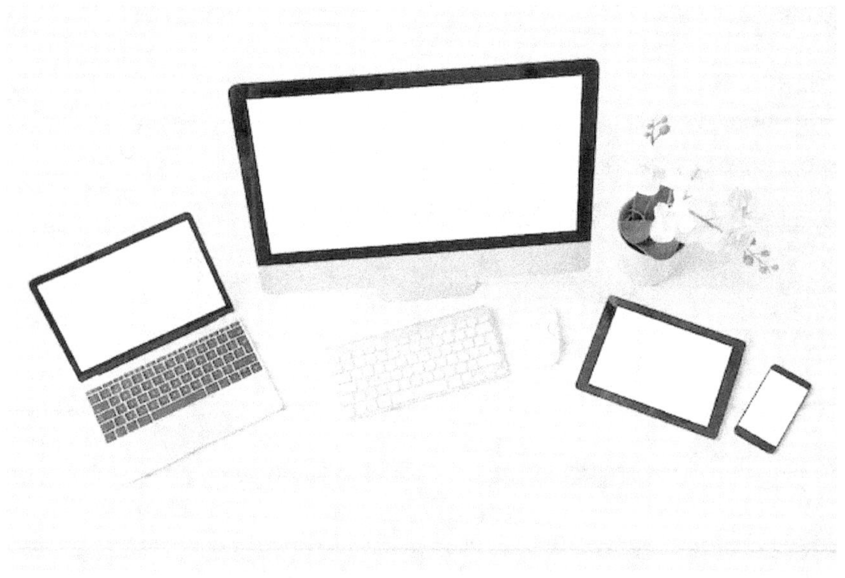

Life in the 21st century consists of screens. Lots of screens! Whether we are at our jobs looking at screens, or relaxing and streaming the latest show. We rely upon spending countless hours looking at screens. I know that I have fallen into the trap of sitting for hours, without a

break while at work, then transitioning to relax on the couch without so much as a walk to stretch out the stiffness.

Like many people, I have been searching for an easy way to transition from a mostly sedentary life, into a life where I have intentional times where I am working out. It is very daunting to start into a program, and even more daunting when you start, and realize that you are nowhere near as in shape as the people in the lessons or videos that you have purchased. You may do well for a week or even a few, but once that initial motivation wears off, what is there to help you with the routine?

This book is meant to assist in building good habits, to help get you past that initial "I can't do it phase" and give you the confidence that you know that you can now carry out a routine. The chapters will be broken down into blocks for breaking down your day and incorporating fitness or stretching routines that can assist in gearing toward a healthier lifestyle, whether you are at work, gaming, or even just relaxing for the evening, this book should in some way speak to you and assist with blocking out your time.

1

Disclaimer

- This book does NOT supersede or replace advice given by a licensed doctor, medical professional, or health advisor.
- This book will primarily focus on exercises, both mental and physical, and stretching prevention and relief.
- This WILL NOT provide:
- List of fitness and productivity applications
- Equipment to assist with fitness
- Cookbook to eat better
- This book WILL provide
- Methods for incorporating fitness into routines
- Methods for improving mental health
- Methods for breaking down mundane activities to allow for sustainable growth
- Stretches and other exercises
- Suggestions on how to incrementally build a healthier lifestyle than the sedentary one you are currently living.

2

Your Routine

How would you define your daily routine? What is your personality, and are you able to pick things up and add them to your routine, or even cut things out completely? When picking up a new task or adding to a routine, it is wise to take a look at things like:

- What are you giving up in order to add this task?
- Do you have time to tackle it in the end?
- Is this something that you will see through until the end?

Many of these questions are hard to assess when you are looking at a new task, especially if you haven't had experience with the given task.

Something that is very hard is to make instant changes that are easy to pick up on, and add to your routine. There is an old saying "if it was easy, anyone could do it." In this instance, you can as well! It will just come with more of an effort on your part. These changes will not come quick, they will take time to do correctly, and overtime, you will notice beneficial changes that will come with consistency and quality repetition.

For our sake, and the sake of this book, we are focusing on fitness and stretching.

CHALLENGE: For a month, take a calendar (I would recommend a PHYSICAL calendar, but phone calendars work just as well), and mark down every time that you do something related to fitness or stretching.

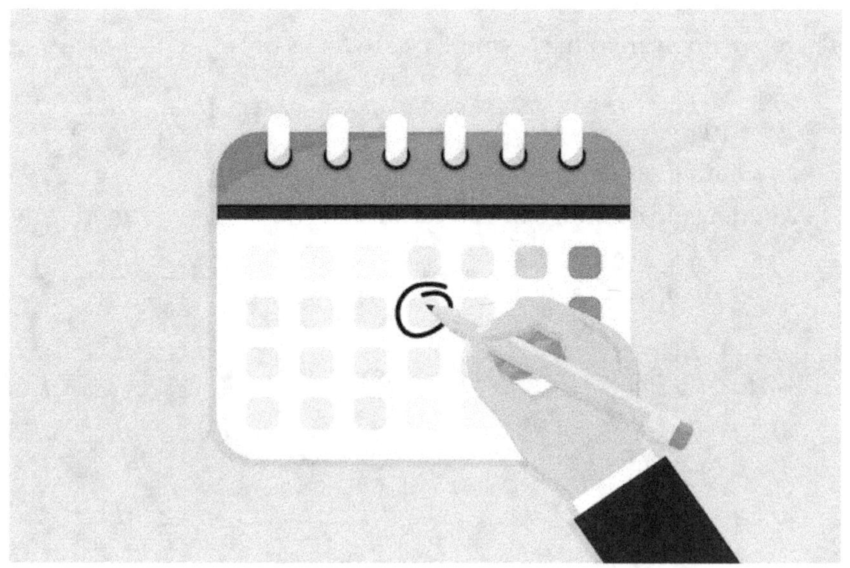

GOAL: At the end of the month, what does your calendar look like? Have you consistently done something that you can look back on and say, "I think I am onto something", or do you see intermittent gaps in your "fitness routine" that you were trying to build.

If you fall into the later portion, you are not alone. There are many reasons why people fail to add to their current routine consistently, even if it is a priority to them. The reason that we will talk about is lack of planning.

Do you have a specific time allocated to be able to allow for you to do your task? I am not saying you need to wake up at 5 am every day, or even workout for 2 hours a day. I am talking about making sure that after your 2 hour meeting block, you schedule time to walk around the office, or do some squats at your desk. Simple tasks that don't require equipment or even draw that much attention.

There are three areas that I would like to focus on:

- At work
- Streaming services
- Gaming (professional or recreational)

At Work:

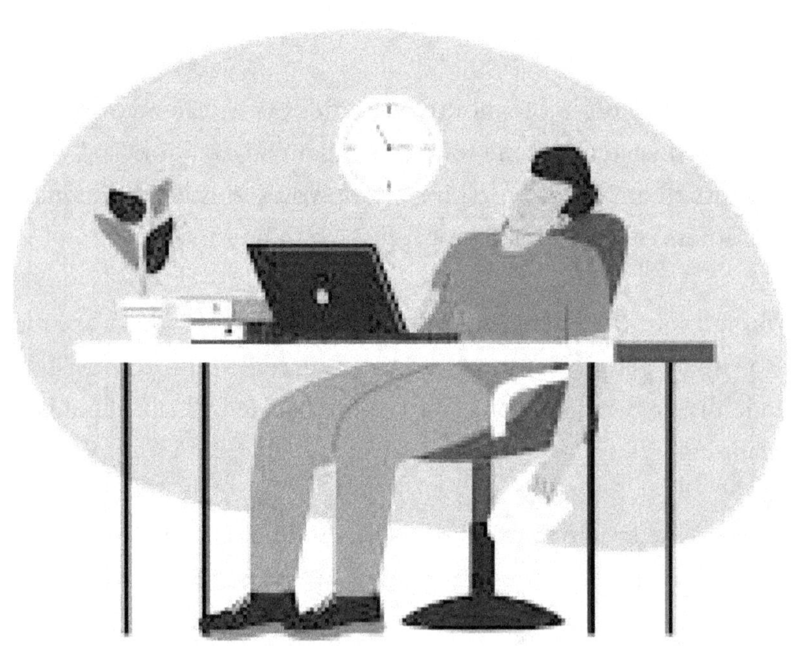

Let's talk about your work routine. You wake up, make your coffee and breakfast, stare at your phone to get your daily news, drive to work (or head down to your basement for your remote job). What is the first thing you do before you log onto your laptop? Try to make associations. This may include when you get to the door, before you go down, do some wall sits, or maybe stretch out your shoulders in the door frame.

So you are now logged on to your computer, now what. You go, answer the countless emails that somehow came in after you logged off last night, you go to your task board, and start getting into your meetings. Many times meetings can go on for hours. I know in my experience, I can sit down for my first meeting at 7 am and as soon as I look up it is time for lunch. Where did the time go, and what did I have to show for all of that time?

Challenge: On Fridays, before you log off for the week, schedule time for yourself throughout the next week. Some days you may not have any free time, or you need to adjust, but place a 15-30 minute break after 2 hours meeting blocks. Intentionally put "mental health break" into the calendar meeting. This way, if people are scheduling their meeting, they know that if they specifically need you during that time, they either have to catch you on the go (adhering to your schedule) or that you will decline their meeting invite and suggest a new time. The more that people work with you, the more they will start knowing and respecting your schedule. You are not only training yourself to respect your time, but also training others to respect it also.

Calendar Etiquette:

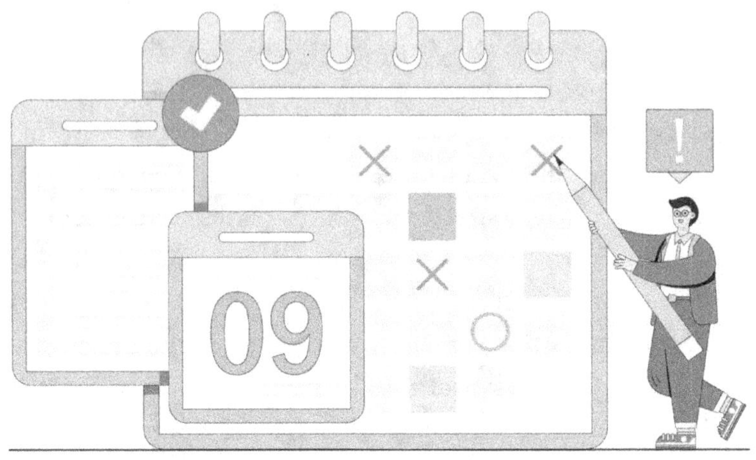

Look for opportunities that you can show your humanness. Can you tell people your dog needs to go out so you need to walk them? People are more willing to accept your breaks if you show that you are human (doing things that they can relate to). Don't just put "busy" or "meeting" in the subject line. To people, these just look like an excuse to get out of something. I have gotten into the pattern of giving specifics like: dentist, doctor, parent teacher conferences. Do I care that I am giving them a portal into my life, possibly, but I know that when they see this, it is more meaningful than just a drop of the hat descriptor in the subject line.

** If this is not a possibility for you, look at the subject matter for meetings, and see if there are meetings where you can be off camera, or even meetings where you don't normally provide input. Can you work in stretches or a walk into that period? Can you take calls on your phone?

Gaming Consoles:

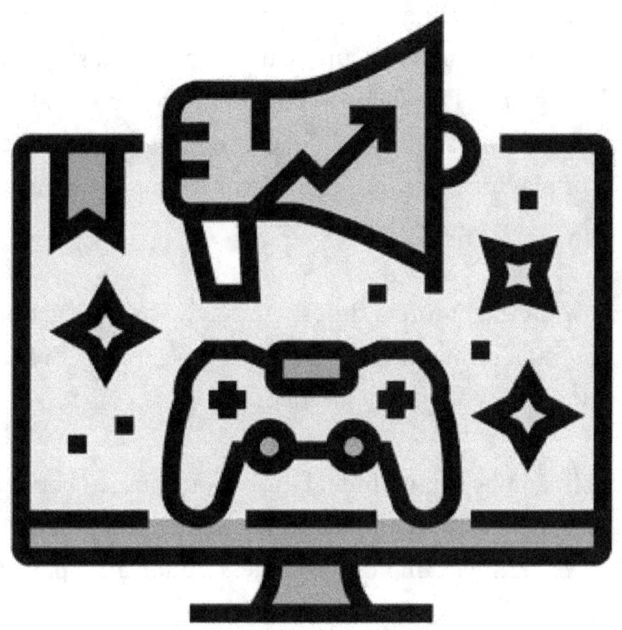

How often have we heard, I will be right up, and that "be right up" turns into two hours later, and you have skipped over the very thing that you were planning. When you are playing a game, how cognizant are you of your time? When you sit down do you say, I will play up until this checkpoint, I will play for an hour, maybe play all night? Do you have a drink and food with you, and is it healthy food? Maybe some of these things apply to you, maybe some of them don't, but regardless of what happens, time seems to fly when you are gaming, especially if it is a game you like.

What are some good ways to break up your gaming? For starters, set an alarm or timer for yourself when you start. Now this will take some self control. There are times that I am better at this than others. Some things that help me are making sure that I have a "hard stop" before I sit down to play a game. This helps to ensure I have a motivation to stop. Other times, I set timers for myself, like finish my drink within the first 30 minutes of playing, at which point I know that I will have to at the very least, get up and go to the bathroom.

What if you want to get into a fitness routine with your gaming? Here are some potential strategies to break up your gaming. Some of these may take some pre-work, some of these can be as you go.

Break spots in games can include: before you start, in between levels, when you fail your task, when you vanquish an enemy, when you have to heal yourself… The examples are endless. Associate a particular area in your gaming with an exercise (i.e. when you die in the game, you have to do 20 push ups. Or when you beat a level, stand up and stretch down to your toes.)

In the following chapters I will have a specific routine built out to address some problem areas that may come along, that will assist in creating a plan to add fitness to your gaming routine.

Streaming Services:
How many of us have gotten the dreaded, "Are you still there?" message as we proceed with the 5th episode of the night? I sure have. I don't know if I am more annoyed that it is asking, if it comes across as

judgemental, or it just makes me look introspectively at myself and tell myself "I should really be doing something productive with my time". All in all, it is not a great feeling. What if I was doing something during these long periods where I had terrible posture at my computer? Could I have broken down the time to add a couch workout, or get up, put in a load of laundry? Of course I could have, but that time has since passed, and I may as well carry on with the tv show right!? WRONG! This is the time where I can make a plan.

Challenge:

Break down the TV show like you would a drinking game. Look at the contents of the show, and add an exercise every time there is a loud bang, or there is a kiss on screen. Between episodes, pause the TV show and do an exercise. Then to reward yourself, continue with the show.

You can also do things while you are watching. Many times you will be at home, or in a more private location, stretch or exercise while you watch the show. Though this may take away from some of the focus of the streaming, it will be adding movement and purpose to your time. (Like you were actually watching as you surf social media)

Things to start being intentional of while you are staring at your screens.

- What do your brakes consist of?
- What are you eating as a snack in between?
- What are you drinking and are you drinking enough water?

Remember to break your time into blocks. Schedule time, set goals, and build in tasks to your routine that are sustainable. Do not make any of these unrealistic or too burdensome that you are overwhelmed just thinking about them. Good habits lead to more good habits! You got this!

3

Motivation

If you are looking at this book, you clearly want to make a change to how you focus your time. From your title, you probably fall into one of those three categories. This is good! Whatever your motivation may be, there are reasons to start pushing for adding fitness into your routine.

Mental:

Mental fitness is a big factor that many people don't take into consideration when they look into why they are losing focus, are losing productivity, are unhappy, or are constantly having unhappy thoughts. Just as athletes exercise and work out, it is just as important for you to be living the way you want to be living. The more you exercise, and care for yourself, the more your mental health will begin to allow you to do the things that you thought were impossible. Again, this growth is little by little, and definitely intentional.

It is often said that people need to improve their mental health, but why? Why is this so important for you? Many times what people don't realize is that their mental health can have a direct impact on how others see you, but so what, who cares how others see you? Regardless of how much we tell ourselves, "it doesn't matter", to some extent there will always be a voice in our heads that "we could have done better", or that we need to be keeping up with the Jones'. Many of these thoughts are very superficial, but they can weigh heavily on our thoughts and minds.

Something that I have been looking into is therapy. For me, I believe that I have a mental block when it comes to therapy. Things that went through my mind are "therapy is only for people with problems", "do I have problems", and "how would therapy really even help me?" Another prohibitor would be cost. Something that I heard on the radio on my way home that I didn't realize is that many companies have programs set up through their benefit packages that allow for a certain number of therapy sessions. Many of these go unused by people that are afforded this luxury. Why is this something that people don't take advantage of? This is a question that I asked myself when listening to this segment. If you have unlimited PTO, have you found what is an acceptable usage during the year? Are you not taking time so that you "look better to your boss?" This can be adding a lot of undue stress to your life. It is easy to get stuck into the rat race of it all.

If you haven't already, read through your HR handbook. Many times, employees will assume that they are getting the most out of their benefits, but they haven't even scratched the surface. According to a study that was published by Amwell (a telemedicine company) "85% of US employee respondents had not used employer-provided mental health benefits" (Golden, 2023). Let me say that again for the people in the back. You may have health benefits that you are paying for, but are not taking advantage of. Some of these difficulties could just be finding the benefits on the company documentation, others could be a failure to understand that their experiences could qualify for coverage, as well as life just getting in the way. Employees nowadays are so busy trying to fit everything into their schedule, climb the corporate ladder, or even just getting from meeting to meeting that their mental health takes a back seat. Some companies are starting to realize this, and are making it mandatory to make advisors available to talk through options whether mental, financial, or career.

Again, take advantage of the things that are offered to you. Sit down and try to fully understand, or reach out to the professionals that are given to you.

Physical:

Go and do a search on why people want to be physically fit. Now I said fit, not jacked, swole, yoked… whatever word you would like to put in there. Fit! Fit meaning healthy, you are okay with yourself from a physical standpoint. Some of these motivations to get physically fit can be: better long term health (paying less later in life for medical), assistance in brain function, better sleep, being able to keep up with your kids or friends. Regardless of the motivation, there are plenty of reasons to keep yourself physically fit. So what is stopping you?

Many people have a mental block that makes it hard to commit to something that doesn't exist in their regular routine. Maybe it is because they bite off more than they can chew, they try to go too hard, too fast and just get frustrated when the hard work doesn't show immediately. Another hurdle that could stop people from adding fitness into their life is they just don't think they have time. We are constantly faced with decisions, whether at work, in a game, or watching the latest TV show. None of these are bad options, but how do we expect to improve ourselves if we never get out of that mundane routine? It is up to us and us alone to build physical activity into our lives.

Some things to look out for that may help to motivate are symptoms that might creep up from being too sedentary. Lethargy can set in and make you restless, and have energy shoot through you in waves. This can affect your mental and physical health. You may start to notice your posture starting to go, you aren't sitting as tall as you once had. Soreness, and shortness of breath. When you get up, do you feel you need to rub your back, or are out of breath just by going up a staircase? These things, compounded with not adding physical activity can be a recipe for troubles in the future. It is important to notice they are happening and take little steps toward modifying your routine.

Bringing in the mental and physical:

Beware of FOMO (Fear of missing out). This can be another potential factor of what is stopping you from adding to your routine. You want to have the latest episode watched so you can talk about it with your friends. Maybe you are gaming with your friends and trying to knock out a campaign, adding anything to your ritual or routine may jeopardize your standing in your friend group or online community. While these are valid, it is also important to remember that no one is going to watch your mental and physical health more than you. Other people do not know what you are going through, or what you need. Stop comparing yourself to these people. We tend to look at the good things in life over the things that cause people trouble. Know that when you contribute to your overall fitness, your overall happiness and self worth will grow with it. This will be noticeable not just to you, but also others, and they will start asking what you are doing to be in this state of happiness.

4

Deterioration

As you age, your body will not always be working for you. There are many ways that your body deteriorates over time that we should draw attention to. One of the best ways to combat this is by keeping your mind and your body strong. Below are going to be a list of common ailments for those that sit a large portion of the day. The main focus will be geared toward those that are sitting at the computer most of the day.

Eyes

I can see just fine! That is not the question we are trying to answer. Will looking at a screen, at work, and at home, affect your overall eye health? One thing to ask yourself is, what is the state of your vision at the moment, and have you noticed a change in the last year, last 5 years, 10 years, etc.?

Check on your eyes. Look for symptoms such as:

- Temporary Blurry Vision

- Dryness in the eyes
- Headaches/Migraines

While mild symptoms such as these may not be a reason for alarm, more studies are taking place to view the effects of screens on our eyes. One such diagnosis is "computer vision syndrome" (American Optometric Association, n.d.). Discussed on the website of the American Optometric Association, they explain that though people have many different tolerances to prolonged exposure to screens, this does not guarantee future issues will not develop. There are things that can be done to assist in strengthening vision, and combat further vision decline.

- Finding the correct lighting
- Improving the lighting of the environment
- Moving monitors to allow for better posture
- Take breaks from prolonged screen exposure
- Allowing for more distance between you and the screen
- REST BREAKS!

Adjusting some things in your environment can assist in working toward protecting your eyes. Once again, a common recommendation is to take breaks from your screen. Just remember, your phone is also a screen, all of us need to understand that screens, while they are everywhere and are necessary for our work, need to have their time, and we need our time away from the screens.

Hands/wrists

Many of the daily activities that we have come to know rely on our hands and wrists. This is a no-brainer, but do we think about them having issues, until they are hurt or are starting to have issues. According to IBISWorld, in 2024, 94% of all US Households have at least one computer. Computers are a way of life, whether it is for work, gaming, shopping, streaming, or managing your finances, we have built a heavy reliance on computers that will only grow into the future (IBISWorld, 2024). It is hard to imagine a future where computers "just go away". Moreover, this calls for us to take action. For current and past usage of computers, a major component of usage is typing.

Hands and wrists can have issues. While many of these issues can look and feel similar, they will have some of the same traits to look out for. Overuse of the hands and wrist that can lead to soreness, pain, swelling, tenderness, and in some cases can lead to surgery. This pain can also be seen in the elbow, forearm. Some common diagnoses include tendinitis and carpal tunnel.

Neck/Back/Shoulder/Spine

Have you ever got up from a long sit, and immediately felt that your back was sore, or you were very tight? What is your first instinct when you feel this? General reaction is to stand up, stretch your arms out, twist right, and twist left. Do you feel that your stiffness or irritation continues to get worse, or that your posture is taking a hit from sitting in a "comfortable position"? You would not be alone in this. Many times, people just attribute this to age, and wear and tear. While this may be the case, the sedentary life may not be helping.

Some potential harms of not focusing on exercising your neck, back, shoulders, or spine can lead to many potential issues. Some of these include:

- Scoliosis
- Deterioration in posture
- Soreness
- Stiffness
- Difficulty standing

All of these warnings and potential diagnosis are things that you should definitely look out for, but just naming these things shouldn't be a scare tactic, but a call to action. In the next chapter we will go over some stretches and exercises that you will be able to do at your desk or at work, that will not disrupt or draw attention to you while you are doing them!

5

Exercises

These exercises that are recommended will be ones that you can do at your desk with little to no equipment. It is important when you are doing these exercises, take deep breaths to ensure there is a proper flow of oxygen.

Eyes

Eye Roll

Sit up straight in your chair. Look straight ahead of you. Without moving your head roll your eyes to the ceiling, in a circular smooth motion roll your eyes to look to the right of you. Smoothly roll your eyes to look at the ground. Continue rolling your eyes to the left, then back up to the ceiling where you started. Do this twice, then take a break.

Blink Break

It is important that your eyes stay well lubricated. Staring at a screen can cause your eyes to start to dry out. Every 15 minutes, take a moment to look away from your screen. Take a deep breath, and blink for 10 seconds.

Place Hands over Closed Eyes

Rub your hands together, to ensure that your hands are warm. Gently place your hands over your eyes. Do not apply too much pressure, but let your eyes feel the warmth from your hands, and relax for 10 seconds.

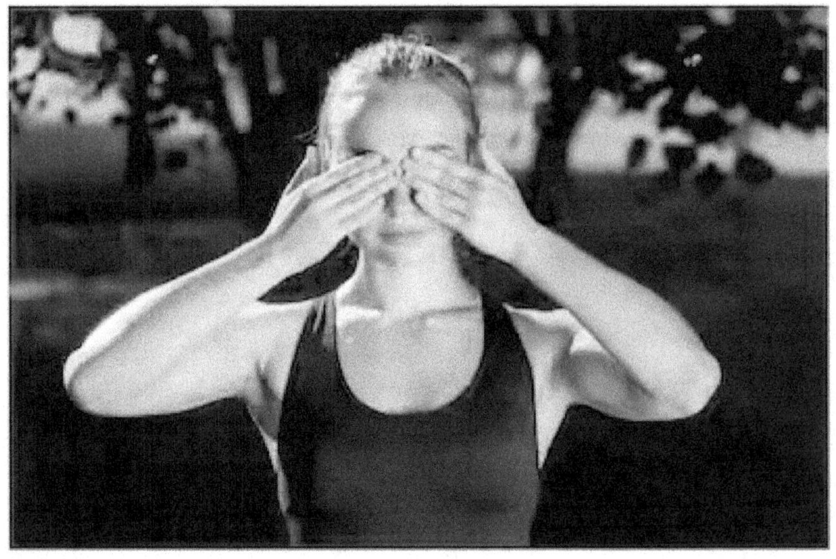

Hands/Wrists

Shake out your hands

This is as easy as it sounds. Loosen your wrists and give it a shake. Do this for a little longer than you feel comfortable. Also, do this throughout your day, as this will allow you to get a flow into your arms, and also allow you to gather your thoughts and give your mind and body a breather.

Hand Waves

Stick your arms straight out with palms facing away from you and fingers up. Move wrists in turning motion like you are waving, or turning a doorknob. Do this 10 times for 3 repetitions.

Grab your hand and pull back

Place your hand in front of you with your fingers pointing up, and your palm facing away from you. Grab your fingers with your other hand, and pull while pushing out with the wrist of the hand that is in front of you. Hold for 30 seconds. You should feel some tension, but don't overdue this to the point where it hurts. Continue doing this as you see fit (Generally 2-3 reps)

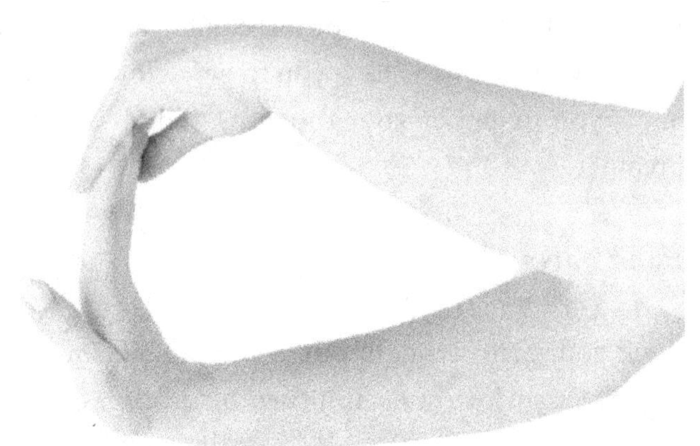

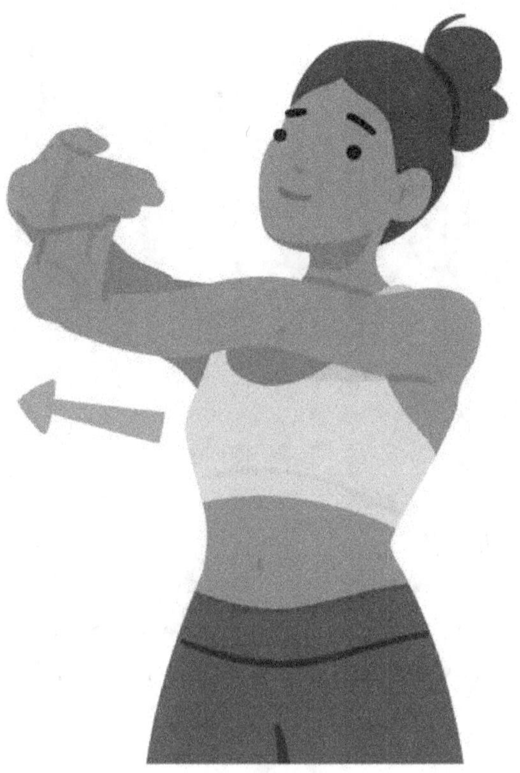

Switch hands and repeat the process with your other hand.

This stretch can be done with your hand facing down or up.

Create a fist with both hands

Place your arms straight in front of you, and rotate your fists in a circular motion. Work with your arms starting loose, and apply more tension little by little. This should not hurt, but you should be able to feel a little bit of pressure.

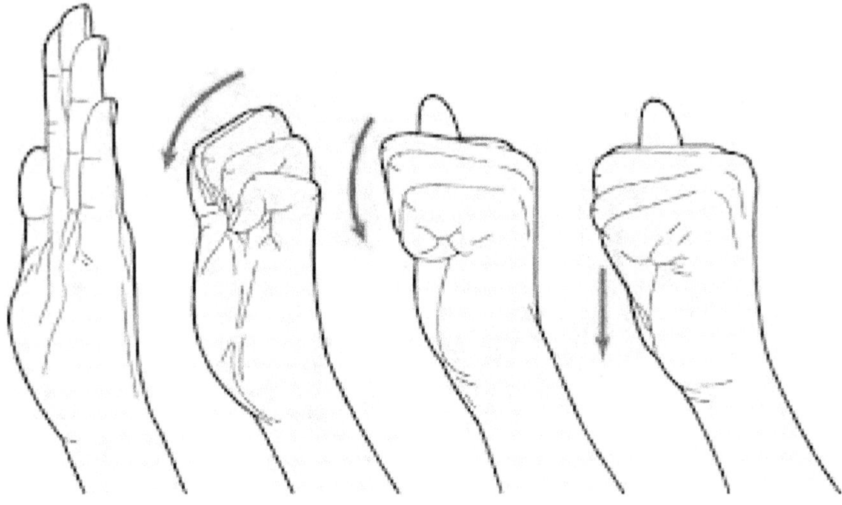

Interlock your hands

Put your hands out in front of you, over a ledge, or over your knees. Rotate your wrists forward and hold for 10 seconds. Repeat for 5 repetitions.

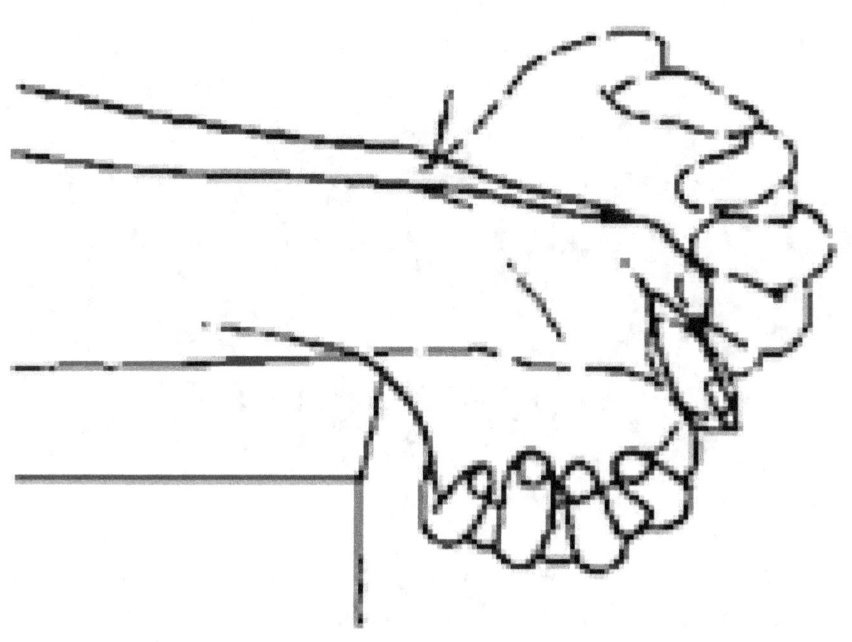

Grab a tennis ball (or some sort of softer ball that has some give)

Squeeze the ball as hard as you can for 5-10 repetitions. Repeat this anywhere from 10-15 times. Do 3 sets of these then stop.

Stretching Hand Up and Pull

Lay the back of your hand onto a table in front of you. Fingers pointing back at you while you apply a little bit of pressure gently lowering your wrist toward your fingers.

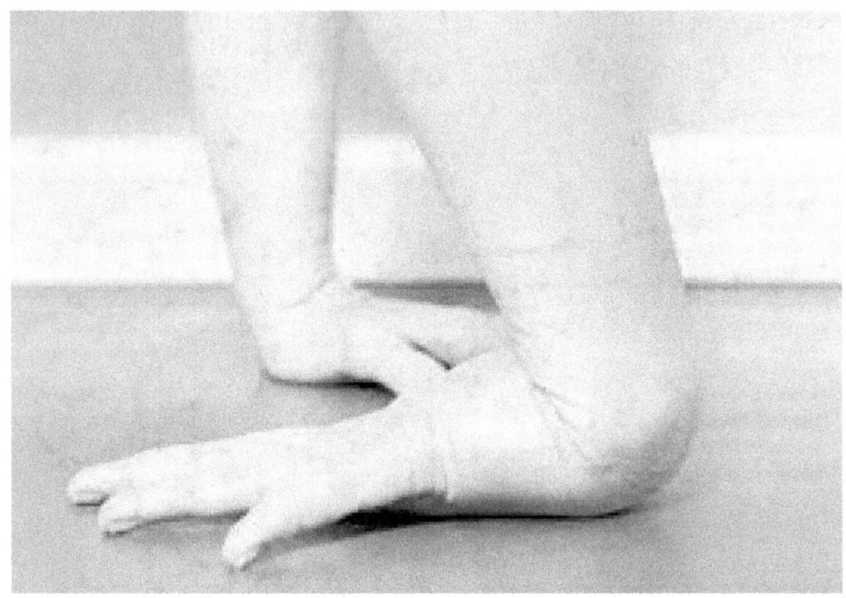

Do not put all of your weight onto your wrist. Ensure that you ease into this motion, as this will create a lot of pressure. Lean slowly until you feel a good stretch, hold for 10 seconds, then release and come up slowly. Do this for 5 repetitions.

Neck/Back/Shoulder/Spine

Look to your Right

Don't strain your neck, but hold when you feel a stretch.

If you are needing more, take your left hand and press against your left cheek. This will apply a little more pressure, and assist in deepening the stretch

Look to the Left

Repeat steps listed above (instead put your right hand on right cheek)

Ear to Shoulder

Do this to the right side then the left.

Bring your right ear to your right shoulder. If you are needing a deeper stretch, use your right hand over your head to assist your ear to your shoulder

Extension of exercise:

Sit down and place your right hand under your leg. Next, bring your left ear to your left shoulder. Hold for 5 seconds.

Feel free to lightly massage your neck and shoulder area as you will now feel that that pull you are creating with your arm underneath you will provide a greater tension.

Head in a circle

Touch your chin to your chest then roll your head to your left. Look up to the sky, and continue rolling your head to your right shoulder. Bring your head chin back to your chest and repeat 5 times.

Repeat the head in a circle exercise above in the opposite direction

Shoulder circles

Sit looking forward in your chair. Sit up straight. Take a deep breath. Roll your shoulders forward 10 times. Next roll your shoulders backwards 10 times.

Hands Behind your head

Sit up straight in a chair. Put your hands behind your head so they cradle your head. Your arm should be pushing your head forward. Push your chest out, and pull your elbows back until you meet resistance. Hold for 10 seconds. Ensure to focus on posture and take deep breaths as this is happening.

Knees/Legs/Feet

Bend Forward

Sit up straight in front of you with your knees in front of you. Lean forward as far as you can. Take your hands and try to grab your toes. Hold this for five seconds. Ensure to breathe in and out on your way up and down. Work every day to get your nose between your knees.

Cross your legs

Take your right leg and cross your left leg where your right ankle lays across your left knee. Push down on your right knee until you find resistance.

Do the same with the opposite leg.

Lean over crossed leg:

While your leg is crossed, lean forward as far as you can. This will help to stretch out the back and leg together.

Knees and feet

If you have the luxury, and can get up and out of your chair. Take a walk and get some fresh air. Not only will this get you away from the things that you have been hitting your head against most of the day, but it will also naturally allow you to release tension and allow you to relax.

Toe Points

Sit in a chair facing forward with your feet flat on the ground. Take your right foot, lift your ankle while keeping your toes on the ground. Push weight into your toes. You will start to feel pressure in your foot and calf. Hold as long as you can.

Do the same thing with your left foot

Add Movement:

At a steady pace bring your heels up one at a time. As one heel goes up, the other heel goes down, all while keeping your toes on the floor.

Leg lift

Sit up straight with your feet flat up on the floor in front of you. Lift your right leg keeping your leg at a 90 degree angle. Lift as high as you can and hold. You will feel tension build. The goal is to get your knee to your chest. If you need assistance, use your arms to pull your knee to your chest.

6

Equipment

I know that at the beginning I said that I will not try to lead you to purchasing a specific product to help assist with issues you may be facing or trying to thwart in the future. This is merely a guide to show different products that are available. Many times, when people are looking for ways to improve, they have to go out and do research on what to buy. This equipment guide will be an assistant for showing how specific equipment can help with your overall strength.

If you have a benefits plan, it is important to look over what you have at your disposal in terms of what is covered for equipment that can assist with improving your health, posture, and productivity (standing desks, ergonomic chairs, feet wedges, and back wedges). Some plans that you should look into are HSA, FSA, health club, access to mental health professionals, and healthy living benefits. Any of these things can be utilized to assist with motivation for building a productive and healthier work environment.

Drink:

Be sure that you are drinking water. This is easier said than done by most people. My little sister is not a water drinker. She hates it. Ensure that if this is you, find ways to increase your water intake, even if it is just one glass per day. While most people can generally drink more water, each person has their limit of water that they should consume. Also, listen to your body. As you drink more liquid, the more you will have to go to the restroom. Some of this can be trial and error, but be sure that you work your drinking of liquids to your schedule. If you know that you have back to back meetings, take a walk 10 minutes before so you can hit the bathroom and also the drinking fountain to refill your drink. Work to find a cadence in consuming liquids that can ensure that going to the restroom doesn't interrupt important meetings, working sessions, and even social breaks.

Even if you are not drinking water, or something healthy, it is still good to get fluids into your system. While drinking "something" is better than drinking "nothing", consider the wear and tear that it will take on your body as a resistance to drinking water can take its toll on your liver, kidneys and other body parts. Doing things now for your health may not be exciting, tasty, or easy. Look at what you can do now as an investment for your future self and health. This also goes for the next point which is "Food". These things can go hand in hand and can be major drivers into how you feel, how you treat others, and how you see yourself.

Food:

EATING IS IMPORTANT. Not eating during the day can bring on many symptoms. Some of these include dizziness, weakness, or fatigue. Eating food on a normal basis, or having snacks available to eat will give you energy and also improve focus. Like drinking too much water, eating too much food can make you start to move slow, become tired, and require

7

Where do we go from here!

- Frequency
- Quality
- Adding walks
- Adding time with pets or family
- Finding a program
- Find a trainer
- Find a therapist
- Go get a physical and see a doctor.
- Finding a gym
- Leave a review for the book
- Sleep!

Now you have a list of things that you can do to move forward to the small changes that you have either implemented, or plan to implement into your routine. None of these things will be a "silver bullet" for curing all that ails you. But if you can make them a habit, you will surely see improvement in not just the physical but also the mental.

These new routines that you have started, what have they done for you? They have helped change your mind that you can stick to something. Sticking with something can lead to a compounding effect of forward thinking. You now think that things are possible that you didn't see before. You now know that if you want something, it won't necessarily come right away. It will take time, hard work, and dedication.

Anyone that is a professional at their craft, they did not just "become" a professional overnight. They constantly practice day after day, have built a routine that works for them, have adjusted that routine to what works for them and the people around them. They have even continued to improve. Even though you may be an "expert" or professional, this does not mean that there won't be new challenges, or things that don't come easily. It means that you have new ways to attack the problems that lie ahead, or deal with the struggle that comes with hardship. Build yourself, day in, day out. Do not expect a fast turnaround. Anything worth getting, takes time. I will leave you with one of my favorite expressions.

"Do not compare your chapter one to someone else's chapter 20".

Remember, implement, and execute! Not everything will be 100% beneficial, but the path to get there will have taught you that you can endure a lot more than you know.

If this book has encouraged you, or proven to be motivational for you, it would be great if you left a favorable review. These reviews will be a guide for books to come in the future. Go and build productive and consistent routines!

RESOURCES:

American Optometric Association. (n.d.). *Computer vision syndrome (Digital eye strain)*. Computer Vision Syndrome. https://www.aoa.org/healthy-eyes/eye-and-vision-conditions/computer-vision-syndrome?sso=y.

Golden, R. (2023, December 1). Why EAPs go unused despite growing mental health awareness. *HR Dive*. https://www.hrdive.com/news/why-eaps-go-unused-despite-growing-mental-health-awareness/701342/

IBISWorld. (2024, August 21). *IBISWorld - industry market research, reports, and statistics*. Percentage of Households With at Least One Computer. https://www.ibisworld.com/us/bed/percentage-of-households-with-at-least-one-computer/4068/